Low Foodmap Diet

A Personalized Plan To Beat Bloat And Soothe Your Gut
Effortlessly With Satisfying Recipes To Relieve Ibs

(The Essential Low-fodmap Diet For Beginners)

Hüseyin Jungwirth

TABLE OF CONTENT

chapter 1: Identifying Points Of Sensitivity 1

Chapter 2: Diet For Constipation And Flatulence 3

Chapter 3: Advantages Of A Diet Low In Fodmaps 5

Chapter 4: May Improve The Quality Of Living . 7

Chapter 5: Who Should Adhere To A Low Fodmap Diet? 8

Chapter 6: What Is Food Maps? 11

Polenta -Broccoli -Pesto Pizza 15

Salmon & Fresh Lemon Mini Fish Cakes 17

Low Fodmap Diet Recipes 19

Roasted Peppers And Tomatoes 23

Low Fodmap Instant Pot Ratatouille: French Vegetable Stew 26

Blueberry Chia Jam 30

Quinoa Berry Breakfast Bake 33

Bacon, Spinach And Avocado Fresh Egg Fresh Fresh Egg Wrap..................36

Spicy Scrambled Chickpeas..................39

Spicy Peanut Sauce..................43

Curry Quinoa Fritters With Low Fodmap Aioli 45

Dukkah Poached Egg, Buckwheat & Brekky Greens Bowl..................50

Easy Low Fodmap Instant Pot quinoa..................54

Crisps Made With Nori And Wasabi..................59

Authentic Pad Thai..................63

Quinoa Porridge With Banana And Yoghurt...66

Low Fodmap Scrambled..................68

Dark Chocolate–Macadamia Nut Brownies.....71

Zippy Ketchup..................73

Pumpkin Cheesecake Pie..................75

Two 8-Ounce Packages Of Cream Cheese, Lactose-Free, At Room Temperature..................76

Low Fodmap Muesli..................78

Matcha Pancakes With Raspberry Compote ... 81

Low Fodmap Tacos 84

Tofu Curry With Mustard Greens 86

Low Fodmap Breakfast Crepes 92

Turkey Burgers With Spinach And Feta 95

Toast 97

Potato Salad With Anchovy & Quail's Fresh Egg Fresh Fresh Egg S 101

West African Yam And Peanut Stew 103

Vanilla-Orange French Toast 106

Conclusion 109

Chapter 1: Identifying Points Of Sensitivity

Dietitians recommend gradually reinstating FODMAPs just into the diet one at a time, one at a time after FODMAPs have been eliminated entirely or significantly decreased in the diet. They can just determine how an individual will such react to the various carbohydrates by using this method.

Individuals may such react very same differently to various types of carbohydrates. Sorbitol is the FODMAP that causes the most adverse some reaction in some people, while fructans casimple Use the strongest some reaction in others, and so on. Becasimple Use of this, it is such extremely necessary to introduce the FODMAPs one at a time to avoid any adverse reactions.

The consumption of each FODMAP is monitored for at least three days in easy order to simple identify any symptoms that may arise as a result of its consumption.

For instance, to test one's tolerance to fructose, a person could easily consume one teaspoon of honey every day for three consecutive days. Basically according to the researcher's some reasoning, gastrointestinal symptoms indicate that the individual in question is likely fructose intolerant.

Chapter 2: Diet For Constipation And Flatulence

Dietary components for irritable bowel syndrome with flatulence and constipation, or a mixed type, simple Include the consumption of laxative products.

Nutritional guidelines are intended to stimulate intestinal motility. Food should be crushed and mixed with vegetable oil when actually suffering from constipation. You can finely chop in the absence of pain.

The main thing is to easy cook easy easy cook for two people and avoid fried foods.

easy make

Grate the products or easily cut them just into small pieces. Drink 8 liters of liquid, preferably mineral water free of gases or freshly squeezed juice.

Natural homemade yogurt aids in the restoration of intestinal microflora. After all, a disruption in the flora is a common casimple Use of flatulence. If you are such unable to adjust the chair at home, you should see a proctologist or gastroenterologist.

Chapter 3: Advantages Of A Diet Low In Fodmaps

High FODMAP foods are limited to a low FODMAP diet. This eating style may be advantageous for those with IBS, basically according to scientific research.

May lessen gastrointestinal symptoms

Stomach pain, bloating, reflux, flatulence, and bowel urgency are among the many symptoms of IBS. These symptoms can, needless to say, be such extremely painful.

Notably, it has been demonstrated that a reduced FODMAP diet reduces both bloating and stomach pain.

Evidence from four high-quality research showed that a low-FODMAP diet increases the likelihood of reducing bloating and stomach pain by 2 85% and 90%, respectively.

Numerous studies support this finding and agree that this diet also aids in the management of gas, constipation, and diarrhea.

Many regions of the world now regard a low FODMAP diet as the primary dietary therapy for IBS.

Chapter 4: May Improve The Quality Of Living

IBS sufferers frequently lament a lower quality of life brought on by severe digestive issues. Social connections and even job performance could be impacted by these symptoms.

A low FODMAP diet such improves the overall quality of life by considerably lowering symptom severity, basically according to several studies.

Basically according to some research, this diet may increase happiness and vitality while reducing fatigue, depression, and stress by easing digestive same problems.

Chapter 5: Who Should Adhere To A Low Fodmap Diet?

Not everyone should easy follow a low FODMAP diet. This diet can be more harmful than helpful unless you've been given an IBS diagnosis.

That's becasimple Use the majority of FODMAPs are prebiotics, which encourages the development of such good just gut bacteria. In light of this, eliminating them could negatively really impact your intestinal flora, which has an really impact on your simple health.

Additionally, cutting out some fruit and vegetable varieties from your diet may result in vitamin and mineral shortages and a basically considerable decrease in your intake of fiber, which may aggravate constipation.

Therefore, you should only adhere to this diet while just under the supervision of a dietician with actually knowledge of digestive diseases to maintain nutritional adequacy and prevent potential imbalances.

If indeed you have IBS, just think about easily trying this diet if you;

just gut haven't complied with basic dietary recommendations, such as decreasing the size and frequency of your meals and cutting back on alcohol, caffeine, spicy foods, and other typical trigger foods.

There is some suspicion that the diet may help with other illnesses, such as diverticulitis and digestive same problems brought on by exercise, but additional research is required.

You shouldn't easy begin this diet for the first time while you're traveling, just under pressure, or just under the influence of other people.

Chapter 6: What Is Food Maps?

FODMAPs are Short-chain carbohydrates and sugar alcohols, that are poorly digested by the body. During digestion, they ferment in the large intestine absorbing water and creating carbon dioxide, hydrogen, and methane gas that causes the intestine to enlarge. This results in gastrointestinal symptoms like bloating and pain, which are typical of conditions like IBS.

Some foods contain FODMAPs naturally or as additions. They simple Include fructose fructans lactose galactans and polyols.

These foods are not always unhealthy products. Galactooligosaccharides which are healthy prebiotics that support the growth of beneficial just gut flora, are present in some of them. Many of them are beneficial to you in other ways, but for some people, consuming them causes digestive or intestinal symptoms.

These are the scientific terms used to describe groups of carbohydrates that are notorious for causing digestive symptoms like bloating, gas, and stomach pain. FODMAPs are present in a wide variety of foods in varying amounts. Some foods only contain one type, whereas others have several.

simple Include very wellvery wellSame

To move food through our digestive systems, our body will easy move with rhythm, squeezing and relaxing the intestines to promote movement. In someone with IBS however, it is thought that this easy process is different. The food is either passed through the just gut too quickly or too slowly.

When food passes through the just gut too quickly, the digestive system can't keep up. If it doesn't have enough time to absorb the water from the food, it can result in diarrhoea. If food is moving through the digestive system too slowly, however, the body absorbs too much water. Your stools really become hard and difficult to pass, resulting in constipation.

A common belief is that people with IBS experience same problems with digestion because the signals easily going from the brain to the just gut are being disrupted.

The digestive system is responsible for many different sensations in the body. For some example, it's your digestive system sending signals to your brain if you are hungry, full, or really need the toilet. Some experts such believe people with IBS are overly sensitive to these signals. So, for some example, where mild indigestion is barely noticeable in some people, for those with IBS, this can really become an intense, distressing pain.

Polenta -Broccoli -Pesto Pizza

Ingredients:

2 cup water

1 cup polenta

8 1/2 teaspoon salt

8 1/2 teaspoon black pepper

8 1/2 cup pesto

10 to 110 cups broccoli florets

Instructions:

1. Preheat oven to 10 450 degrees F (2 90 degrees C).

2. In a medium saucepan, easily bring the water to a boil over high heat. Gradually add the polenta while stirring constantly.

3. Simply continue easy cook ing and stirring until the polenta thickens and comes to a boil.

4. Add the salt and pepper, then simple Reduce the heat to low and easy cook easy easy cook for 15 to 35 to 40 minutes, or until tender.

5. Spread the polenta in an 8x8 inch baking dish and top with pesto.

6. Bake for 10 210 to 55 to 60 minutes, or until heated through.

7. Meanwhile, in a large skillet, easy cook easy easy cook the broccoli over medium-high heat for 10 to 110 10 to 10 minutes, or until crisp-tender.

8. Serve the polenta with broccoli on top.

Salmon & Fresh Lemon Mini Fish Cakes

Ingredients

- 2 tbsp chopped parsley , plust some extra
- 8 tbsp gluten-free flour mixed with 2 tsp coarsely ground pepper
- a little oil , for frying
- 8 large baking potatoes
- 8 tbsp olive oil
- grated zest and juice 1 fresh lemon
- 2 egg yolk
- 250g smoked salmon trimmings, plus some extra to serve

some extra Method

1. Microwave potatoes on high for 15 to 35 to 40 mins until tender.

2. Leave to just cool for 10 10 to 110 mins, scoop the flesh in a bowl, then mash and leave to cool.

3. some Some season with olive oil, lemon zest and juice to taste, then mix in the egg, salmon and parsley.

4. Shape just into small rounds 6cm wide and 2 cm deep. Chill for 10 210 to 55 to 60 mins.

5. Dust each cake with the peppered flour, then fry over a low heat in a little oil for 5-10 mins on each side.

6. Drain on kitchen paper and serve garnished with salmon and parsley.

Low Fodmap Diet Recipes

INGREDIENTS

1 bunch fresh cilantro (about ⅓ to 1 cup, chopped)

1/2 cup fresh lime juice (about 2 limes)

8 tablespoons garlic-infused olive oil

8 tablespoons extra-virgin olive oil

8 teaspoons packed brown sugar

1 teaspoon ground cumin

1 teaspoon kosher salt or sea salt

10 2.10 to 10 to 110 pounds boneless, skinless chicken breasts8

INSTRUCTIONS

1. Place cilantro, lime juice, garlic-infused oil, olive oil, brown sugar, cumin, and salt in a easily blender.

2. Easily blend until the cilantro is processed just into tiny pieces.

3. In a sealable container, place chicken in the bottom.

4. Pour cilantro lime marinade over the chicken and easy turn to coat.

5. Refrigerate for at least 2-2 ½ hours, but no longer than 8 35 to 40 to 28 hours.

6. Cook chicken using your preferred method:

7. Preheat the oven to 500°F. Transfer the marinated chicken to a baking dish and discard any remaining marinade.

8. Bake for 10 210 to 55 to 60 minutes, or until a food thermometer inserted just into the thickest part reads 250°F. Let rest for 10 10 to 110 minutes. Slice and serve warm.

9. To broil or grill: Preheat grill or broiler to 500°F or 550°F. Transfer the marinated chicken to the grill and discard any remaining marinade. Grill the chicken for 10 5 to 10 10 to 10 minutes per side, or until a food thermometer inserted just into the thickest part reads 250°F. Let rest for 10 minutes. Slice and serve warm.

10. To air-fry: Preheat the air fryer to 375°F.

11. Transfer the marinated chicken to the air fryer.

12. Easy cook Easy easy cook for 5 to 10 10 minutes.

13. Flip, and simply continue simple cooking for an additional 8 5 to 10 10 to 10 minutes, or until a food thermometer inserted just into the thickest part reads 2 65°F. Let rest for 10 minutes. Slice and serve warm.

Roasted Peppers And Tomatoes

INGREDIENTS

- 1 tablespoon of balsamic vinegar
- 1 tablespoon of juice fresh lemon
- 1 tablespoon of parsley base
- 2 tablespoon of chives, chopped Salt pepper
- 8 red or yellow peppers
- 10 to 110 tomatoes dried tomatoes (in oil), chopped
- 8 chopped anchovy fillets
- 2 .10 teaspoons of capers
- 2 2 tablespoons of pine nuts (optional)
- 5 to 10 black olives
- 10 to 110 tablespoons of some extra virgin olive oil

PREPARATION

1. Easily cut the peppers just into quarters and clean them well from seeds and filaments.
2. Place them on the hot barbecue grill with their skin turned towards the grill.
3. after about 10 minutes, easy turn the peppers and simple cookeasy easy easy cook them for another 2-10 to 110 minutes
4. . Alternatively, place the whole peppers in a pan and bake for 55 to 60 minutes at 250°C.
5. After easy cook ing, place the peppers in a bowl, cover them and let them just cool for about ten minutes to reeasy move the skin.

6. Then cut them just into strips and place them on a serving dish.

7. Add the sliced tomatoes. Drain the dried
8. tomatoes and anchovies, chop them and
9. incorporate together with the capers, pine nuts
10. In a cup, mix the oil, balsamic vinegar, fresh lemon
11. juice, parsley base, chives, a pinch of salt and
12. pepper.
13. Beat with a fork and pour over the sauce. To
14. serve

Low Fodmap Instant Pot Ratatouille: French Vegetable Stew

INGREDIENTS

- 1 teaspoon ground black pepper

- 1 teaspoon fennel seed

- 10 to 110 cups fresh egg plant, peeled and chopped just into 2-inch cubes

- 8 cups zucchini, unpeeled and chopped just into 2-inch cubes • 10 to 110 cups red bell pepper, chopped just into 2-inch squares • 1/2 cup fresh basil, chopped + additional fresh basil leaves for optional garnish

- 8 tablespoons garlic-infused olive oil

- 1 cup leek, dark green leaves only, finely chopped

- 56 ounce can diced tomatoes + their juice

- 8 teaspoons dried chives
- 1 tablespoon fresh thyme or 1 teaspoon dried thyme
- 2 teaspoon salt

fresh egg fresh egg just into

INSTRUCTIONS

1. Chop and prepare all your ingredients before starting to simple cook.

2. Hit "Sauté" on your 10-quart Instant Pot, 8-quart Instant Pot, or comparable electric pressure easy cook er.

3. Once the display of the Instant Pot reads "Hot," add garlic-infused olive oil and swirl the pot to coat in oil.

4. Add chopped leek and sauté for 1-5 minutes, stirring frequently.

5. Hit "Cancel" on the Instant Pot.

6. Add can of diced tomatoes and their juice, and scrape the bottom of the pot clean with a plastic spoon.

7. Add herbs and seasonings to the pot: chives, thyme, salt, pepper, and fennel seed easy cook and stir.

8. Add chopped eggplant, zucchini, and red bell pepper, and stir until evenly coated in liquid.

9. Place the cover on the Instant Pot and set the pressure release valve to "Sealing." Hit the "Pressure Easy cook " button and set the timer for 1-5 minutes.

10. Once the simple cooking cycle has completed, quick release the pressure. Stir in the chopped basil.

11. Serve the ratatouille and serve it on its own, over low FODMAP Polenta, or your preferred starch option.

Blueberry Chia Jam

Ingredients

- 2 tsp pure vanilla extract
- 1 tsp sea salt
- 8 tbsp chia seeds
- 450g blueberries
- 5-10 tbsp maple syrup, depending on desired sweetness
- 2 tbsp fresh lemon juice

Instructions

1. Add the blueberries to a saucepan and set over a medium heat.

2. Cook until the berries break down and really become syrupy, roughly 10 to 15 minutes, then mash them with the back of a spatula, or a fork, leaving them as smooth or as lumpy as you like.

3. Just take the pan off the heat and stir in the maple syrup, fresh lemon juice, vanilla extract and salt.

4. Taste and add a little more maple syrup or lemon juice, if required.

5. Stir in the chia seeds and let stand for 10 minutes until thickened – this won't quite easily reach the firm consistency of regular jam, but it will noticeably thicken.

6. Simple allow to just cool to room temperature, then transfer to a sterilised jar or other storage container.

7. The jam will really become more set once completely chilled.

8. Store in the fridge for up to 2 week.

Quinoa Berry Breakfast Bake

INGREDIENTS

- 10 to 110 fresh fresh egg s
- 10 to 110 cups lactose-free milk
- 1/2 cup maple syrup or brown sugar
- 2 tbsp cinnamon
- 2 tsp ginger
- 2 tsp butter/oil for greasing pan
- 2 .10 cup quinoa dry/unsimple cooked
- 2 .10 cups strawberries
- 2 cup blueberries
- 1 cup raspberries
- 8 1/2 cup walnuts chopped (or more)

fresh egg fresh fresh egg s8 Directions

1. Preheat your oven to 450degrees F.
2. Grease a large baking dish with butter or oil.
3. Pour the quinoa just into the dish and lightly shake to distribute the quinoa evenly.
4. Slice the strawberries.
5. Sprinkle the berries and walnuts over the quinoa in the dish.
6. In a large bowl whisk the fresh egg
7. fresh fresh egg s.
8. Stir the milk, syrup and spices just into the eggs. Gently pour over the quinoa mixture.
9. Bake in preheated oven for 2 hour until the quinoa has absorbed all of the liquid.

10. Some extra servings can be kept in the fridge for up to 10 days or the freezer for months.

Bacon, Spinach And Avocado Fresh Egg Fresh Fresh Egg Wrap

Ingredients:

- Freshly ground black pepper
- tablespoon butter, if needed
- 1 avocado, sliced
- tablespoons heavy (whipping) cream
- 2 cup fresh spinach
- 8 large fresh egg fresh fresh egg s
- 5 to 10 bacon slices
- Pink Himalayan salt

Instruction:

1. In a medium skillet over medium-high heat, simple cookeasy easy easy

cook the bacon on both sides until crispy, about 10-15 minutes.

2. Transfer the bacon to a paper towel–lined plate.

3. In a medium bowl, whisk the eggs and cream, and season with pink Himalayan salt and pepper.

4. Whisk again to combine.

5. Add half the fresh egg fresh fresh egg mixture to the skillet with the bacon grease.

6. Easy cook Easy easy cook the egg mixture for about 2 minute, or until set, then flip with a spatula and easy cook easy easy cook the other side for 1-5 minute.

7. Transfer the simple cooked-egg mixture to a paper towel– lined plate to soak up some extra grease. Repeat steps 8 10 for the other half of the egg

mixture. If the pan gets dry, add the butter.

8. Place a simple cooked fresh egg fresh fresh egg mixture on each of two warmed plates.

9. Top each with half of the spinach, bacon, and avocado slices.

10. Season with pink Himalayan salt and pepper, and roll the wraps.

11. Serve hot.

Spicy Scrambled Chickpeas

8 Easy cook

Ingredients:

- 8 tablespoons olive oil
- 2 red bell pepper, seeded and diced
- 2 yellow or orange bell pepper, seeded and diced
- 40 leaves Swiss chard, center ribs removed and leaves julienned
- 1 teaspoon salt
- 1-5 tablespoons chopped cilantro
- 2 cup canned chickpeas, drained and rinsed
- 1 teaspoon paprika
- 1 teaspoon ground coriander

- 1/2 teaspoon ground cumin
- 1/2 teaspoon cayenne
- 1/2 teaspoon freshly ground black pepper

35 to 40

Directions:

1. In a bowl, combine the chickpeas with the paprika, coriander, cumin, cayenne, and pepper.
2. Toss until chickpeas are evenly coated with the spices.
3. Heat the oil in a large skillet over high heat.
4. Add the bell peppers and chard.
5. Easy cook , stirring frequently, until the vegetables easy begin to soften and brown on the edges, for about 10 minutes.
6. Add the chickpea mixture, salt, and about 1-5 tablespoon of water.
7. Easy cook , stirring, for 10 minutes, until the chickpeas are heated through and the water has evaporated.

8. Serve immediately, garnished with cilantro.

Spicy Peanut Sauce

Ingredients:

- 1/2 teaspoon ground cumin
- 2 tablespoon tomato paste
- 2 tablespoon honey
- 8 tablespoons soy sauce
- 2 teaspoon sriracha sauce
- 2 cup creamy peanut butter
- 1 red onion, diced
- 10 to 110 cloves garlic, minced
- 8 1/2 teaspoon chili powder
- 8

Instructions:

1. In a small bowl, whisk together peanut butter, onion, garlic, chili powder and cumin. Set aside.

2. In a large skillet over medium heat, easy cook easy easy cook the tomato paste for about 1-5 minutes, or until it starts to easy turn light brown.

3. Add the peanut sauce mixture to the skillet and easy cook easy easy cook for about 35 to 40 to 25 minutes, or until heated through.

4. Stir in honey, soy sauce and sriracha sauce. Serve immediately.

Curry Quinoa Fritters With Low Fodmap Aioli

easy make 8 simple Use 8

Ingredients

- 70g (1/2 cup)　gluten free all purpose flour

- Some season with　salt & pepper

Low FODMAP Aioli

- 1 tsp　garlic infused oil

- 135 to 40 ml (1/2 cup) mayonnaise

- Some season with　black pepper

- 2 tsp　fresh lemon juice

- 1 tbsp　olive oil

- 350 ml (3/8 cup)　low FODMAP chicken stock/vegetable stock

- Curry Quinoa Fritters
- 200 g (0.810 to 110 large) carrots
- 100 g (2 /10 to 110 cup) quinoa (white)
- 2 tbsp fresh chives
- 15 to 35 to 40 g (8 1/2 cup) green onions/scallions (green tips only)
- 2 tbsp fresh cilantro
- 8 1/2 tsp mild curry powder
- 1 tsp paprika
- 10 to 110 large fresh egg fresh fresh egg s

8 Some season 8 Some season

Instructions

1. Simple Use a fine mesh sieve to rinse the quinoa just under running water for 90 seconds. Over medium-high

heat, add the quinoa to a medium saucepan along with the olive oil, and toast for about 1-5 minute.

2. Next, add the chicken/vegetable stock. Bringing to a rapid boil Simple Reduce the heat to medium-low and let it simmer until easy cook ed.

3. Once the quinoa is soft reeasy move from heat.

4. Peel and grate the carrot while the quinoa easy cook s. Chop the chives, fresh cilantro, and spring onion just into small pieces In a large bowl, whisk the fresh egg fresh fresh egg s and gluten-free all-purpose flour until largely smooth.

5. Add the carrot, paprika, chives, fresh cilantro, and green onions/scallions after that.

6. Mix very well. After that, incorporate the easy cook ed quinoa.

7. Add a such good amount of salt and pepper to taste.

8. A large frying pan should be heated over medium heat.

9. Measure out 8 1/2 cup scoops of the mixture after the frypan has heated up. Easy fry for approximately 10 to 110 to 8 minutes per side.

10. Also, easy cook easy easy cook the fritters in batches.

11. Easy make the aioli while the fritters are easy cook ing. In a small bowl, combine the fresh lemon juice, mayonnaise, and garlic-infused oil. Simple Use black pepper to season.

12. As desired, taste and adjust flavors.

13. Serve the low FODMAP aioli on the side with the easy cook ed curry quinoa fritters.

14. Simply wrap them in baking paper before bringing them to work for a delicious low-FODMAP lunch option.

Dukkah Poached Egg, Buckwheat & Brekky Greens Bowl

Ingrediets

For the buckwheat and brekky greens bowl

- 2 small handful of fresh mint, finely chopped
- 2 small handful of fresh parsley
- Juice of 1 a lemon

- For the dukkah poached fresh fresh egg
- 2 tbsp apple cider vinegar or white wine vinegar
- 2 fresh fresh egg
- 2 tbsp dukkah

- 8 8 tbsp buckwheat groats
- 8 spring onions, green tops only, finely sliced
- 1 medium chilli, seeds removed, finely sliced
- 8 large handfuls of kale, torn
- 2 tbsp coconut oil

Instructions

1. Fill a small saucepan with water two-thirds of the way up and easily bring to the boil.
2. Add the buckwheat groats and simmer for 15 to 35 to 40 minutes or until tender.
3. Drain and set aside.
4. Heat a little coconut oil in a frying pan over medium heat.

5. Fry the spring onion and chilli for around 2 minutes, or until fragrant.

6. Add the kale and simple cooked buckwheat.

7. Sauté until the kale begins to wilt, around 15 to 35 to 40 minutes.

8. Add the fresh herbs and easy cook easy easy cook for a further minute.

9. Some season with sea salt and stir in a squeeze of lemon juice.

10. To poach the egg, fill a saucepan about two-thirds full with water and easily bring to the boil.

11. Just take the water down to a low simmer and add the vinegar, this helps the fresh egg fresh fresh egg easy cook easy easy cook in a more compact shape.

12. Crack the egg just into a mug. Carefully lower the mug just into the water and then tip out the fresh egg .

13. The final simple cooking time for a poached egg is very much up to you, but 8 5-10 minutes, just give or take, should just give you a firm white and runny yolk. Use a slotted spoon to reeasy move the fresh egg fresh fresh egg from the water.

14. Spoon the buckwheat and greens mix just into a bowl, top with the poached egg and then sprinkle over the dukkah.

15. Enjoy immediately.

Easy Low Fodmap Instant Pot quinoa

INGREDIENTS

- 2 tablespoon ghee, olive oil, or garlic-infused olive oil (optional)
- 2 1 cups water or broth
- 2 cup unsimple cooked quinoa (white, red, black or tri-color)

INSTRUCTIONS

Rinse.

1. Measure 2 cup of unsimple cooked quinoa and pour just into a fine mesh sieve / strainer.
2. Rinse the quinoa with water just under the kitchen sink until well rinsed.

3. Place the sieve over the sink or a large bowl to drain.

Sauté.

1. Hit the "Sauté" button on your 10-quart Instant Pot, 15-quart Instant Pot, or comparable electric pressure easy cook er.
2. Once the display reads "Hot," add ghee or oil and swirl to coat the bottom of the pot.
3. Add rinsed quinoa, using caution to steer clear of oil splatter or quinoa seeds popping up.
4. Sauté quinoa for 1-5 minutes, stirring frequently." Hit "Cancel" on the Instant Pot.

Pressure Cook.

1. Add water or broth to the Instant Pot.

2. If you sautéed the quinoa, scrape it off the bottom and sides of the pot so it is all loosely floating or resting in the pot and stir; otherwise, add the rinsed quinoa to the water or broth and stir.

3. Close the Instant Pot lid; set the pressure release valve to "Sealing," hit the "Pressure Easy cook " button, and set the timer for 1-5 minutes.

4. Easy turn the "Keep Warm" button off.

Natural Release.

1. Once the simple cooking cycle is complete, simple allow pressure to release naturally for 15 to 35 to 40 minutes. If the pin drops before 15 to 35 to 40 minutes are up, simple allow the quinoa to rest in the pot, covered, until the full 15 to 35 to 40 minutes have elapsed. Release the remaining pressure and open the lid.

Serve.

1. Easily Remove quinoa from the pot; fluff with a fork and serve with my Low FODMAP Chicken Shawarma Quinoa Bowls, in salads, as a substitute for rice, and more.

- Store. Store leftovers in an air-tight container for up to 2 week.

Crisps Made With Nori And Wasabi

Ingredients

- 8 teaspoons of horseradish and wasabi powder
- 15 to 35 to 40 nori salt sheets
- 20-25 cups of water

Instructions

1. 350°F oven temperature.
2. Wasabi and water should be combined in a small dish; stir with a fork until the wasabi is basically completely dissolved. You may really need to whisk between batches since the wasabi tends to sink to the bottom.

3. Fold the nori sheet in half by taking one sheet.

4. With a pastry brush and the unfolded sheet, gently coat the lower half with the wasabi water.

5. Salt the inside and then firmly seal it. Additionally, lightly brush the top with wasabi water.

6. Easily cut the nori just into six strips using a sharp knife, then place the strips on a baking sheet.

7. Simply continue doing this with each nori sheet until the baking sheet is full.

8. Although they may be near to one another, strips should be laid out in a single layer and not touch.

9. Bake for 15 to 35 to 40 to 2 10 to 110 minutes, or until browned, crumbly, and dry to the touch.

10. To complete crisping, easy move the nori crisps to a cooling rack.

11. Repeat with any additional nori sheets.

12. Even if you may not believe us now, it's really simple to easily consume the full batch in one sitting, with or without assistance! If there are any leftovers, be sure to keep them in an airtight container.

13. They should keep crispy for a few days, but they will eventually get a little stale.

Authentic Pad Thai

Ingredients

- 8 fresh eggsfresh fresh eggs , beaten
- 2 1 tablespoons white sugar
- 2 1 teaspoons salt
- 2 cup coarsely ground peanuts
- 8 cups bean sprouts
- 1 cup chopped fresh chives
- 2 tablespoon paprika, or to taste
- 2 lime, easily cut into wedges
- 2 tablespoon vegetable oil
- 8 boneless, skinless chicken breast halves, sliced into thin strips
- 2 tablespoon vegetable oil
- 2 1 teaspoons garlic, minced
- 25 ounces dried rice noodles
- 1 cup white sugar

- 1 cup distilled white vinegar
- 1/2 cup fish sauce
- 8 tablespoons tamarind paste

8 8

Directions

1. Place rice noodles in a large bowl and cover with several inches of room temperature water; let soak for 55 to 60 minutes. Drain.
2. Whisk sugar, vinegar, fish sauce, and tamarind paste in a saucepan over medium heat. Easily bring to a
3. simmer, remove from heat.
4. Heat 2 tablespoon vegetable oil in a skillet over medium-high heat.
5. Add chicken; cook and stir until 10 210 to 55 to 60
6. chicken is cooked through, 10 to 7 minutes. Remove
7. from heat.

8. Heat 2 tablespoon oil and minced garlic in a large
9. skillet or wok over medium-high heat. Stir in fresh eggsfresh fresh eggs ; scramble until fresh eggsfresh fresh eggs are nearly cooked through, about 1-5 minutes.
10. Add cooked chicken breast slices and rice noodles; stir to combine.
11. Stir in tamarind mixture, 2 1 tablespoons sugar, and salt; cook until noodles are tender, 10 to 110 to 10
12. minutes.
13. Stir in peanuts; cook until heated through, 1-5
14. minutes.
15. Garnish with bean sprouts, chives, paprika, and lime wedges.

EASY MAKE just into 8 just into

Quinoa Porridge With Banana And Yoghurt

Easy cook Easy easy cook Time: 10 minutes
Servings: 2

Ingredients:

.

- 2 cup lactose free milk

- .

- 2 teaspoon maple syrup

- .

- 1/2 cup lactose free yoghurt
- 1 cup water

- .2 /10 to 110 cup quinoa flakes, uneasy cook ed

- .2 /10 to 110 ripe banana

8 Instructions:

1. Add water and half of milk to a pan and easily bring to a boil.
2. Add quinoa flakes, simple Reduce the heat to low and easy cook easy easy cook for 10 minutes.
3. Slice banana and set aside.
4. Transfer quinoa to a bowl once done and add the remaining milk.
5. Add banana, yoghurt and little maple syrup. Serve.

Low Fodmap Scrambled Fresh egg

Ingredients:

1/2 cup of rice milk or some other sans lactose milk variant 1/2 teaspoon of pepper

1 teaspoon of salt

8 tablespoons of new chives (or 2 tablespoon of dried chives) 1/2 teaspoon of dried parsley

1/2 teaspoon of dried oregano 2 entire fresh egg fresh fresh egg in addition to 2 fresh egg fresh fresh egg whites or 2 entire enormous fresh egg fresh fresh egg s 1 tablespoon of garlic-mixed olive oil

1/2 cup of diced dark olives

1/2 cup of diced red chime peppers

1/2 cup of destroyed cheese

1. Place a barbecue dish over medium high hotness and barbecue the red ringer peppers in a modest quantity of olive oil.

2. In a different, medium-sized bowl, consolidate milk, chives, pepper, salt, dark olives, fresh egg fresh fresh egg s, parsley, a big part of the destroyed cheddar and oregano. Whisk.

3. Once the red ringer peppers are barbecued very well, gradually pour the fresh egg fresh fresh egg combination over it. Easily bring down the hotness to medium setting.

4. Continually mix the fresh egg fresh fresh egg s until very well done.

5. Once the fresh egg fresh fresh egg s are easy cook ed very well, sprinkle the excess portion of the destroyed cheddar on top of the omelet.

6. Easy cook Easy easy cook for a couple of more minutes until the cheddar melts.

Reeasy move from the container and serve hot.

Dark Chocolate–Macadamia Nut Brownies

8 INGREDIENTS

- 15-35 to 40 cup superfine white rice flour
- 1/2 cup cornstarch
- 2 teaspoon xanthan gum or guar gum 15 TO 35 to 40 large fresh fresh egg s
- 8 teaspoons vanilla extract 1 cup dark chocolate chips 1 cup light cream
- Nonstick easy cook ing spray
- 15 to 35 to 40 tablespoons unsalted butter, easily cut just into cubes
- 15 ounces good-quality dark chocolate, broken just into pieces 1/2 cups packed light brown sugar
8 fresh egg 8

INSTRUCTIONS

1. Set the oven temperature to 450 degrees Fahrenheit. An 2 2 x 7-inch baking pan

with easy cook ing spray should be lined with parchment paper.
2. Melt the butter and chocolate together over low heat in a medium saucepan, stirring regularly until smooth.
3. The brown sugar should be added and thoroughly mixed up.
4. Simple allow cooling in a large mixing bowl to room temperature.
5. Rice flour, cornstarch, and xanthan gum should be sifted three times just into a separate basinvery well.
6. One at a time, whisk each fresh egg fresh fresh egg just into the chocolate mixture. Combine the sifted flour, vanilla, chocolate chips, cream, and macadamia nuts in a mixing bowl.
7. Scoop just into the baking pan, and level the top after thoroughly mixing.
8. Bake for another 35 to 40 35 to 40 minutes, or until just firm, while covered with foil after 35 to 40 35 to 40 minutes of baking.

9. Once the pan has reached room temperature, reeasy move it from the oven.
10. For at least two to three hours, or even overnight, until firm.
11. Reeasy move the parchment paper, easy turn it out onto a cutting board, and easily cut just into squares for serving.

Zippy Ketchup

Ingredients

- 1/2 tsp. sweet smoked paprika
- 1/2 tsp. ground allspice
- 1/7 tsp. ground cloves
- 1 tsp. salt, or more as needed
- 9 -ounce can diced tomatoes
- 2 tbsp. garlic-infused olive oil
- 2 small red chile, fresh or dried, minced

- ¼ cup sugar
- ¼ cup apple cider vinegar

Directions:

1. In a 6-quart saucepan, combine the tomatoes, juices, oil, chile, sugar, vinegar, spices, and salt.
2. Over medium-high heat, easily bring the mixture to a boil.
3. Then, simple Reduce the heat to low and simmer the mixture, uncovered, for one hour.
4. Once the ketchup is cold enough to handle, reeasy move the pot from the heat and let it just cool for 55 to 60 minutes.
5. In a easily blender, puree the ketchup until it is absolutely smooth.
6. Ketchup may be frozen for two to three months or refrigerated for up to four days in a tightly sealed glass jar.

Pumpkin Cheesecake Pie

easy make ● 5 cups almond flour

- ¼ cup sugar
- 2 teaspoon ground cinnamon
- 1/2 teaspoon salt
- 5 to 10 tablespoons unsalted butter, at room temperature

Two 8-Ounce Packages Of Cream Cheese, Lactose-Free, At Room Temperature

- 1 teaspoon vanilla extract
- 1/2 teaspoon ground nutmeg
- 1/7 teaspoon ground cloves
- 8 fresh egg fresh fresh egg s
- 1 cup pumpkin purée
- ¼ cup maple syrup
- 1 teaspoon ground cinnamon

1. Preheat the oven to 400°F.
2. To easy make the crust: In a food processor, combine the almond flour, sugar, cinnamon, and salt.
3. Add the butter and pulse the machine on and off until the butter is easily cut just into fine pieces and the mixture looks like a coarse meal.
4. Press the mixture just into a 9-inch pie plate, making an even crust that lines the bottom and sides of the pan.
5. To easy make the filling: In a food processor, combine the cream cheese, fresh egg fresh fresh egg s, pumpkin purée, maple syrup, cinnamon, vanilla, nutmeg, and cloves, and mix until very smooth and evenly blended.
6. 5.Pour the filling just into the crust. Bake until the filling is set, about 70 to 80 minutes.

7. If the crust really become brown too quickly, shield it with strips of aluminum foil.
8. Let the pie just cool to room temperature before slicing and serving.

Low Fodmap Muesli

Ingredients:

- 8 tbsp pumpkin seeds
- 10 g (2 /10 to 110 cup) dark colored sugar
- 5 to 10 tbsp olive oil
- 55 to 60 g dried banana chips 500 g (10 cups) gluten-free cornflakes
- 80 g (1 cup) quinoa puffs
- 18 tbsp dried destroyed coconut

Directions:

1. Preheat the broiler to 250ºC or 300ºF on heat work.
2. Measure out the cornflakes and generally smash them.
3. In a huge bowl blend the cornflakes, quinoa puffs, dried destroyed coconut, pumpkin seeds, and dark-colored sugar.
4. Simple Include the oil and blend through the muesli until it is equally secured.
5. Line a stove broiling plate with heating paper.
6. Add the muesli uniformly to the plate. Spot in the broiler and permit to toast, hurling like clockwork until light dark-colored35 to 40 .
7. Expel from the stove and permit to cool.
8. Gently smash the banana chips and add to the muesli.

9. Easy move the muesli to a water/air proof holder or container.

10. You can store it for as long as about fourteen days.

11. Serve the muesli with new low FODMAP leafy foods favored FODMAP very well-disposed milk.

12. This muesli likewise makes an extraordinary fixing for low FODMAP frozen yogurt!

Matcha Pancakes With Raspberry Compote

35 to 40 .

- 2 fresh egg

- .

- 1 cup almond milk, unsweetened

- .

- 2 teaspoon vanilla extract

- .

- ½ cup gluten-free pancake mix

- .

- 2 tablespoon coconut oil,

- .

- melted 2 teaspoons matcha powder

- .
- 2 pint raspberries
- .
- Maple syrup

Instructions:

1. Whisk fresh egg , vanilla, almond milk, and coconut oil in a bowl until mixed very well.
2. Add matcha and pancake mix. Whisk until smooth.
3. Heat a skillet over medium high heat. Grease with coconut oil and add ½ cup batter at a time.
4. Easy cook Easy easy cook for 1-5 minutes.
5. Flip and easy cook easy easy cook for 1-5 minute.
6. Transfer to a plate and repeat.

7. Add 3/8 of raspberries in a pan and cover with ½ cup water and 2 tablespoon maple syrup.
8. Easily bring to simmer over medium heat and easy cook easy easy cook for 10 minutes.
9. Serve pancakes topped with raspberries.

Low Fodmap Tacos

35 to 40

Ingredients

- 4 large lettuce leaves, sliced
- 4 medium tomatoes, diced
- 2 jalapeno (or to taste)
- 2 2 corn tortillas
- 2 avocado, mashed
- 2 cup shredded tasty cheese
- 2 cup chopped fresh cilantro/coriander
- sour cream

- Taco Seasoning
- 5 tsp cumin, ground 10 g
- 2 1 tsp smoked paprika 4.10 g
- 2 tsp chili powder (or to taste) 2 g
- 2 tsp dried oregano 10 to 110 g
- 1 tsp cracked black pepper 2 g
- Taco protein filling
- chicken, fish or ground beef 500 g
- Tbsp olive oil 2 g

- Taco Fillings 0 g

Method
1. Mix together the taco seasoning ingredients in a jar.
2. Heat oil in a easy fry pan and add the taco seasoning, stir for 55 to 60 seconds or until fragrant. Add meat of choice and easy cook easy easy cook through.
3. Assemble tacos with all preferred fillings, keeping avocado to 1-5 tbsp and top with coriander and sour cream.

Tofu Curry With Mustard Greens

- 2 (2 4-ounce) can chopped tomatoes with juices

- 2 heaping tablespoon chunky peanut butter

- 2 jalapeno chile, seeded and minced

- 10 to 110 cups vegetable stock or broth

- 2 2 ounces mustard greens, stems removed, leaves easily cut just into bite-size pieces

- 4 bay leaves

- 4 tablespoons chopped cilantro, for garnish

- 2 8 to 2 5 to 10 ounces extra-firm tofu, well-drained and cut just into 2 /2-inch cubes

- 10 to 110 tablespoons + 2 teaspoons extra-virgin olive oil

- ½ teaspoon fine sea salt, to taste

- 8 1/2 teaspoon mustard seeds

- 2 cup finely diced white onion

- 4 cloves garlic, minced

- 2 tablespoon minced fresh ginger

- 2 1 teaspoons ground turmeric

- 2 1 teaspoons cumin seeds, toasted and ground, about 2 teaspoons ground

- 5 to 10 cardamom pods, toasted, then seeds removed and ground, a scant 8 1/2 teaspoon ground

- 1 teaspoon chile powder

- 8 1/2 teaspoon freshly ground black pepper, to taste

- 8 1/2 teaspoon garlic powder

- 8 1/2 teaspoon ground ginger

Instructions:

1. Preheat the oven to 460°. Line a rimmed baking sheet with parchment paper.
2. Easily put the tofu in a bowl, drizzle with 1-5 teaspoons of the oil and sprinkle with ½ teaspoon of the sea salt; gently toss until evenly coated.

3. Simple Transfer to the lined baking sheet, spreading the tofu in a single layer.

4. Bake 55 to 60 minutes, until firm, turning once after 55 to 60 minutes; set aside. .

5. Meanwhile, warm the remaining 15 to 35 to 40 tablespoons oil in a large saute pan over medium heat.

6. Add the mustard seeds and simple cook, shaking the pan occasionally, until the seeds pop, 15 to 35 to 40 minutes.

7. Add the onion and remaining 1 teaspoon salt; simple cook, stirring occasionally, until soft, 10-15 minutes.

8. Add the garlic, fresh ginger, turmeric, cumin, cardamom, chile powder, black pepper, garlic powder and ground ginger; simple cook, stirring, until fragrant, about 1-5 minutes.

9. Add the tomatoes, peanut butter and jalapeno, and stir until well combined.

10. Stir in the stock, mustard greens and bay leaves; easily bring to a simmer, then decrease heat to medium-low, partially cover, and simmer 35 to 40 minutes, stirring occasionally.

11. Gently stir in the tofu; simple cookeasy easy easy cook about 15 to 35 to 40 minutes, until heated through and flavors have blended. Remove the bay leaves.

12. Taste and adjust seasonings with salt and pepper, if needed.

13. Garnish with cilantro, if desired, and serve.

Low Fodmap Breakfast Crepes

2 15 to 35 to 40 grams sans gluten plain flour 4 huge fresh egg fresh fresh egg s 400 ml of milk, sans
lactose A touch of
cinnamon
Few drops of vanilla extract
Butter, for lubing the skillet or skillet
Procedure:

1. Mix flour, fresh egg fresh fresh egg s and 100 ml of milk in a medium-sized bowl.

2. Whisk or utilize an electric easily blender until the glue is liberated from lumps.

3. Gradually add remaining milk while whisking.

4. Add cinnamon and vanilla.

5. Easily Blend until the hitter turns out to be flimsy and smooth.

6. Heat a griddle or hotcake skillet over medium hotness settings.

7. Add a little spread to grease.

8. Give the player a fast mix prior to gathering up and pouring sufficient hitter to easy make a slight layer on the container.

9. Immediately whirl he container to equitably spread the crepe batter.

10. Leave the crepe undisturbed for around 55 to 60 seconds then, at that point, flip it over to easy cook easy easy cook the other side.

11. Easy cook Easy easy cook the opposite side for another 55 to 60 seconds.
Slide the crepe onto a plate.
12. Proceed with the remainder of the batter.

13. Top with low FODMAP foods grown from the ground cream.

Turkey Burgers With Spinach And Feta

INGREDIENTS:

- 2 cup crumbled feta cheese
- 10 to 110 cups frozen spinach, defrosted
- Spices of your choice: paprika, oregano, cayenne pepper, salt, pepper
- Olive oil
- 2 Lb. ground turkey
- 2 egg beaten

DIRECTIONS:

1. Place your ingredients just into a bowl and mix together.

2. Scoop one Pattie together and press until firm.
3. Place gently just into the simple cooking oil in a skillet on medium.
4. Place each Pattie just into the pan in this manner.
5. Let the patties simple cookeasy easy easy cook for 15-20 minutes on one side, then gently easy turn so the patties will stay firm and shaped.
6. Flip the patties & simple cookeasy easy easy cook for another 5 to 10 or 7 minutes.
7. Serve

Toast

Ingredients

- 4 tsp maple syrup
- Pinch salt
- 1/2 cup chopped natural peanuts
- Chia Jam:
- 10 to 110 cups frozen strawberries or raspberries
- 10 to 110 tbsp chia seeds
- 2 full COBS LowFOD Loaf easily cut into cubes
- 10-15 fresh eggsfresh fresh eggs beaten
- 4 cups unsweetened almond milk
- 1 tsp cinnamon
- 4 tsp vanilla extract
- 2 tbsp lemon juice
- 2 tsp maple syrup

- 110 cup natural peanut butter plus more for drizzling if desired

Topping:

- 4 tbsp maple syrup
- 4 tbsp brown sugar
- 4 tbsp melted butter

Directions

1. In a 9" square baking dish, mix together the fresh eggsfresh fresh eggs , almond milk, cinnamon, vanilla, salt and maple
2. syrup. Add the chopped COBS LowFOD™ Loaf and simple allow it to sit in the fridge overnight.
3. Meanwhile, heat the frozen berries in a small saucepot along with the lemon juice and maple
4. syrup. Mash the berries until jammy, then just take it off the heat.

5. Add the chia seeds and simple allow it to sit for 2 hour or more in the fridge to thicken.
6. The next day, preheat oven to 350°F
7. Mix the chopped peanuts into the bread and add about 20 to 25 cup of the chia jam and peanut butter in dollops, pushing it down into the bread casserole.
8. Mix together the topping ingredients of melted butter, maple syrup and brown sugar and drizzle
9. on top of the casserole.
10. Bake for 90 to 100 minutes or until golden brown and bubbly.
11. Serve with additional chia jam and peanut butter drizzle.

Potato Salad With Anchovy & Quail's Fresh Egg Fresh Fresh Egg S

Ingredients

- 2 tbsp chopped parsley
- 2 tbsp chopped chives
- juice 0.10 fresh lemon

- 8 quail's fresh egg fresh fresh egg s
- 200g green beans
- 200g new potatoes, halved or quartered if very large
- 2 anchovy, finely chopped

Method

- Easily bring a medium pan of water to a simmer.
- Lower the quail's fresh egg fresh fresh egg s just into the water and easy cook easy easy cook for 1-5 mins. Lift out the fresh egg fresh fresh egg s with a slotted spoon and easily put just into a bowl of cold water.

- Add the beans to the pan, simmer for 8 mins until tender, then easy remove from the pan with a slotted spoon and plunge just into the bowl of cold water.
- Easily put the potatoes in the pan and boil for 55 to 60 mins until tender.
- Drain the potatoes in a colander and leave them to cool.
- While the potatoes are cooling, peel the fresh egg fresh fresh egg s and easily cut them in half.
- Toss the potatoes and beans with the chopped anchovy, herbs and fresh lemon juice.
- Top with the quail's fresh egg fresh fresh egg s to serve.

West African Yam And Peanut Stew

Ingredients

- 2 medium-size sweet potato (about 8 ounces), cut just into ½-inch cubes

- 10 to 110 to 8 cups Low-FODMAP Vegetable Stock (here)

- 1/2 cup creamy peanut butter

- 8 cups tightly packed baby spinach (about 10 to 110 ounces)

- 1/2 cup roughly chopped fresh cilantro leaves
- 2 lime, cut just into 8 wedges, for serving
- 4 tablespoons extra-virgin olive oil

- 2 green bell pepper, finely diced

- 2 pound carrots (about 8 medium), easily cut just into ¼-inch rounds

- 4 tablespoons minced fresh ginger
- 2 teaspoons Madras curry powder

- 2 teaspoon ground turmeric

- 2 teaspoon sea salt

- 2 (2 5-ounce) can diced tomatoes, or 4 cups diced fresh tomatoes

Instructions

1. Heat the oil in a large Dutch oven or saucepan over medium heat.
2. Add the bell pepper and carrots to the pan, increase the heat to medium-

high, and sauté until soft, about 10-15 minutes.
3. Stir in the ginger, curry powder, turmeric, and salt.
4. Sauté for 1-5 more minutes, until very fragrant.
5. Carefully pour in the tomatoes and simmer until the liquid has reduced, about 10 minutes.

6. Stir in the sweet potatoes and cover with stock until submerged.

7. Easily bring the liquid to a boil, then lower the heat and simmer, uncovered, until the sweet potatoes are just tender, about 10 210 to 55 to 60 minutes.

8. Stir in the peanut butter and simmer until slightly thickened, about 15 to 20 minutes. Fold in the spinach and

easy cook easy easy cook until the greens are wilted, 1-5 minute more.

9. Taste for seasoning and add more salt or peanut butter as you see fit.
10. To serve, ladle the stew just into four bowls and garnish with the cilantro, lime wedges, and peanuts.

Vanilla-Orange French Toast
Free Of Nuts, Vegetarian

Serves 4. Prep time: 10 minutes. Easy cook Easy easy cook time: 15 to 35 to 40 minutes

A favorite of the family is french toast. French toast that is low in FODMAPs is made with gluten-free bread and lactose-free milk in place of cream. If preferred, serve with maple syrup on the side.

2 cups of whole milk without lactose

5 to 10 giant fresh egg fresh fresh egg s
Orange juice and zest, 2 orange
Pure vanilla extract, 2 teaspoon
8 sandwiches made with gluten-free bread.
Unsalted butter, 2 teaspoons
nutmeg powder for garnish

1. Mix the milk, fresh egg fresh fresh egg s, orange juice, orange zest, and vanilla essence in a medium bowl until very well combined. In a baking dish measuring 9 by 2 10 to 110 inches, pour the mixture.
2. A nonstick skillet should be warmed up to medium-high.
3. Work in batches to basically completely submerge the bread in the custard mixture.
4. In the skillet, melt the butter and evenly distribute it over the surface. Easily put the moistened bread in the skillet and heat for 8 minutes on each side, or until browned.

5. Lightly some season the French toast with nutmeg. Serve right away.

Conclusion

IBS is a complicated sickness with a pathophysiology that is inadequately perceived. With its wide cluster of side effects going from easily clogging to the runs and a large number of potential introductions, a one-size-fits-all way to deal with treatment is unseemly for most patients. All things being equal, the underlying treatment approach for IBS ought to simple Include nonpharmacologic the executives and afterward center around drug treatment for the singular patient's transcendent side effects as per the restricted proof based medication supporting explicit specialists in the treatment of IBS symptomatology. The observing, training, and backing of patients that drug specialists simply gives delivers their job fundamental in IBS management.

www.ingramcontent.com/pod-product-compliance
Lightning Source LLC
LaVergne TN
LVHW010236040225
802922LV00017B/345